****

The Art

of

Internship

****

Sean L. Sawh M.D.

Francy M. Sawh M.D.

About the authors

Sean L. Sawh M.D.

Sean graduated from University College Dublin, Ireland and completed his Surgical Internship at the Harvard Program in General Surgery, Brigham and Women's Hospital in Boston, Massachusetts. He was subsequently offered an inter-residency robotic fellowship in Urology at Henry Ford Hospital in Detroit, Michigan before moving to the University of North Carolina at Chapel Hill where he is now a senior Urology resident.

Francy M. Sawh M.D.

Francy completed her medical school training in 2009 at Ross University School of Medicine. She worked at the University of North Carolina at Chapel Hill as part of the Pediatric Intensive Care Unit program before taking up a position as an Anesthesiology resident.

TABLE OF CONTENTS

INTRODUCTION

Wayne Newton gives a great story about Frank Sinatra. Evidently, Frank was supposed to perform at a Philadelphia concert one night. Frank was late and the owner was getting nervous so he climbs onto the balcony on the second floor of the building to see if he could see Frank coming. It was a rainy night, and across the alley-way, he sees a taxi cab come to a stop. Frank bolts out of the cab, and runs pell-mell down the alley in the rain. When he gets close to the stage door, Frank stops, takes off his wet coat, hangs it over his shoulder, straightens his hat, lights a cigarette, and calmly strolls onto the stage.

Now what does Frank Sinatra, rain and cigarettes have to do with Medicine? It's simple. The story here is learn to be calm. If you train yourself to stop and think, and prepare yourself before you walk into any situation, you will do your job better, and will ultimately dispense better patient care.

This is not a book to teach you how to work up a fever. This is not a book that teaches you how to come up with differential diagnoses or what tests to order in a given scenario. This book will not help you with USMLE, ABSITE or any other exam. There are many books like that out there and you should be familiar with at least one of them.

Internship, like all of Medicine, is an art. This is the book that you can read to help you prepare for Internship year in terms of how to plan your day, and basically, how to do your job effectively and be an invaluable member of your team. If this book is skewed toward a surgical internship, it is because of my own bias. But the principles are universal and can be helpful to anyone in any Internship anywhere. Consider this light reading to teach you how to handle what will ultimately be one of the most challenging years in your medical or surgical career. The aim is to erase some of the misconceptions about Internship that many students face as they transition from final year medical student to Intern. This aim is to also aid Foreign Medical Graduates who come to the United States after medical school and may not have had the same exposure to the duties of a U.S. medical school student.

Rule #1: Don't lie

It may sound simple, but when your facing a senior resident, chief resident or Attending who asks you if you did or did not do something, and you know that if you tell the truth you may get yelled at, your primordial instincts return, and your first reaction is to protect yourself…so you may be tempted to lie. This is a mistake that can potentially cause more harm than you can possibly imagine, as you will no longer be a trusted member of your team.

In my first week of Internship, on my Birthday of all days, I was sent to consent a patient for a surgical procedure. The patient asked me what time she could expect to be taken to the OR. It was a Saturday, and I recalled that my chief resident had mentioned to the Attending that they would take the patient to the OR later than afternoon. What I had not realized was that the chief was referring to another patient at a different hospital. I consented my patient and informed her that it would be some time before we took her to the OR. About three hours later, my chief resident pages me and asks me to come to the patient's room to meet with him and the Attending. The patient can no longer be taken to the OR because she apparently ate breakfast when I told her that she would not go to the OR for several hours. The patient was a "frequent flyer" and knew that she had enough time to eat breakfast that day since it would be more than six hours before we took her to the OR. My chief turns to me and asks if I told the patient that we would not be taking her to the OR for several hours, therefore giving her the OK to eat her breakfast. I stood there paralyzed. The chief, who was not exactly known for his kind demeanor, glared at me. The Attending was muttering several curses and incantations as the case would now be delayed. So, I lied. I stood there and lied.

It must have been the way I said it, or just my body language, but the chief knew that I was lying. He took me outside and proceeded to scream at me (which in retrospect was unacceptable of him by the way) for causing the case to be delayed and for lying. He let me know that I was now untrustworthy, and that my lies had placed a great burden on the team as they now had an untrustworthy Intern, and that my every assignment would have to be checked and re-checked by someone else on the team. I was devastated. Here I was, a brand new Intern, and I had now broken the cardinal rule. I could potentially have been ruined as I would have had the reputation of being a liar and therefore someone who could not be trusted.

I could see where the chief was coming from. Everyone on a team has an assigned duty. If you can't do your job properly, then that means that someone else on the team has to do your job in addition to theirs, which leads to more work for someone else. Lying makes you un-trustworthy, and a liability to your team. In my case, I was fortunate in that as it turned out, one of the nurses who witnessed what happened to me later called the chief resident and told him that the patient had already eaten prior to my ever coming to consent her, so the case would have been delayed anyway. The chief was decent enough to call me and apologize for screaming at me. The Attending had screamed at him, so he was displaying some characteristic displacement behavior by now screaming at me. The chief reiterated the importance of never telling a lie, as the consequences of lying will be far worse than the consequences of whatever you were trying to cover up in the first place. We could have taken that patient to the OR at any time later that day, but my trustworthiness would have been shattered forever.

I am reminded of a fellow intern who would routinely make up his own vitals on a patient. In our hospital, we were supposed to physically walk to every patient's bedside and get their vitals out of the nursing chart. It was a real pain to do it, as the charts were never where they were supposed to be. So this guy decided that for midnight vitals and lab values, he was just going to copy the last set of vitals and labs on the list, which would have been at least twelve hours old and of course, quite useless. He just changed the numbers by a fraction to ensure that nobody noticed what he was doing. It worked for him for a few weeks, until one morning when we found a post-operative patient with a creatinine of 2.3, up from his previous value of 0.9. The chief was suspicious, and double checked every lab and vital sign on the list in front of the intern. On discovering his scheme, he checked the lists for the past several nights when that intern was on-call, and discovered that this was a routine modus operandi for this intern. Now, while this guy was not fired, the schedule was changed so that he was forced out of the surgical rotations and sent to rotate with other services where he would do pure scut work, and where there was a Physician's Assistant who could essentially cover all of this guy's duties to ensure that he basically was not needed on the team. He is no longer a resident at that hospital. Don't lie. It will ruin you.

Rule #2: Trust no one. Assume nothing.

Now this rule sounds a bit harsh, but it will serve you well if you stick to it. While it does create more work for you, it will ensure that you do your job well, and will ultimately result in better patient care.

Another anecdote to illustrate this rule is as follows. While I was getting the inputs and outputs from patients one night, I could not find the chart for Mrs. Castro, a 65F who had a nephrectomy for renal cell carcinoma. The nurse in-charge of her was on a break, so I continued to round with the intention of coming back to see that patient. Unfortunately, I forgot, and decided to telephone the nurse's station to find out the Ins and Outs on that patient. The nurse was still missing in action, but the nurse that I spoke with told me that she knew for a fact that the patient had put out 200cc of urine over that 6-hour shift, which was pretty much within normal limits from my point of you. While waiting for rounds at 6am, Mrs. Castro's nurse called me to let me know that the patient had indeed made zero urine over the past twelve hours. I was dumbfounded. Here was someone who had failed to do her job by not recording or noticing that her patient had made zero urine over an entire shift. But she was not the only one guilty of not doing their job. I was also guilty. Had I looked at the chart like I was supposed to, I would have seen that no urine outputs were recorded, and I would have made it my business to find that nurse and get the necessary information. Instead, I trusted someone who was not even covering that patient. This resulted in that patient ending up in the ICU in acute renal failure.

There are many stories like that when you are told something by someone that turns out to be untrue. Remember, this is your job and these are your responsibilities. Look at that X-Ray yourself. Read that pathology report yourself. Examine that patient yourself. Trust no one. Assume nothing.

Rule #3: Find the Diamond.

In medicine, and particular, in general surgery, you will come across someone who you simply will dislike as they will speak to you very rudely. They will be very painful to work with as a result of their abrasive personality. A part of you will simply detest them as they will make your already stressful life even more unpleasant.

On one particular rotation, I was being berated on a daily basis by a chief resident who was known for his prolific writing skills, keen surgical instincts, but more so, for his horrendous personality. Every intern that worked with him hated this guy. In fact, most every resident that I knew simply detested him. But the program loved him as he was good at his job, and everyone just accepted that they had to work with him.

After another session in which he assured me that I was the most incompetent Intern that he had come across in his seven years as a resident, I was moping in the cafeteria eating some meat of indeterminate origins (our cafeteria special). One of the Cardio-Thoracic Surgery Fellows who was also known for his brilliance that was eclipsed only by his kindness, came to sit with me and noticed my dejection. It was only my third month of internship, so I was still pretty shaky in the grand scheme of things. Eventually, I confessed to this Fellow what was bothering me, and asked him for his advice on how to handle my temperamental chief.

The Fellow gave me this lesson, which I have found to be one of the most invaluable pieces of advice that I have ever received. "Find the diamond", he said to me. "Let me break it down for you like this. There are many, many different attitudes and personalities that you will come across in this career, and unfortunately, you're going to find more than a handful of people who simply have horrible attitudes. But, here's what you need to do. When these people are yelling at you, bear in mind that there is an invaluable piece of advice in what they're telling you. It's like having a 3-carat diamond buried in a pile of cow dung. It may just all seem like an unpleasant mess at first, but if you search through what they're saying, and learn to ignore the insults and the way that they are addressing you, you will learn something from them that will serve to make you a better doctor overall. These are not stupid people. They're just unpleasant people. Find the diamond in the dung that they are giving you. Learn from every opportunity regardless of how unpleasant it may seem at first glance. Find the diamond".

Rule # 4: All pages are equal.

Now at first glance, this rule is somewhat misleading. Naturally, a page about a patient whose hemoglobin has dropped by 6 points is far more important than the occasional page that you will get about the patient wanting a sleep aid. This rule is based on the advice imparted by a visiting professor one cold Wednesday night.

I was on the Urology service and we were having a guest lecture come and speak to us at our Wednesday night grand rounds. The lecturer was one of the most respected radiation oncologist in the world and even has his own set of criteria named after him. We sat there expectantly, awaiting the invaluable pearls of wisdom that he would cast before us, surely revolutionizing the way we practiced. He came in, introduced himself by his first name to us all, and took the time to ask each of us our first names. He then stood in front of the room, and informed us that we would now be privy to the most important lecture that we had ever heard, and would ever hear for the rest of our career. There were audible snickers at this somewhat boastful remark, but by the end of the lecture, it was clear that there was truth to this grandiose claim.

"Of all the pages you will get, the most important page that you can receive on a daily basis, is the page from your significant other. You may have work responsibilities, but you also have social or family responsibilities. You must therefore return any page, or rather, text message that you receive from your significant other in a timely fashion. Your work is not your life, and if you let it become that way, then you have failed". We sat there dumbfounded. We were expecting some sort of clinic pearl, but what we were getting here, was so much more important.

This man was absolutely right. In our busy, hectic schedules, we must remember that the people in our lives play a vital role in our well-being. They are the ones who support us when we come home after a tough day. They are the ones who listen to us when we are down. They are also going through Intern year albeit with a different flavor. Make time for that other person or persons in your life. Return their text message when you can. Let them know that they are as important to you as your job. At the end of the day, they're the ones that love you. Respect them and return their messages when you can.

Rule #5: Load the Boat.

Yes, you have made it. You've passed countless exams, quizzes, tests etc. You're finally in residency. But, bear in mind that this does not mean that you are the all knowing master of your specialty. You are an intern. You have only just begun your training, so if you get called to make a decision on a patient, or to give advice on a consult, or if you are unsure in anyway of something, load the boat. That is, don't be the only one on the team who knows something. If things go badly and something happens to a patient because you failed to act or made a bad decision, then the blame falls on you. However, if you seek the advice of a senior resident, or at least let them know what's going on, if the things do go wrong, you will not be the only one held responsible for what happened.

Many new interns seem to think that they are the ones who should make any decision presented to them, even though they are somewhat unsure of what to do. You will not be viewed as being weak if you ask a question. Remember, first and foremost in any residency, you are not expected to know everything. Indeed, you are not expected to know anything. But, you are expected, to learn quickly.

Load the boat. Make sure that you are not the only person involved. If you are not sure, ask someone.

Rule #6: Don't stop the train.

If a patient is going to the OR that day, or going to get a CT-scan, or is going to get a transfusion or any other such plan, do everything in your power to ensure that you don't do something that prevents this procedure or test from happening. That is, make sure you get everything in place to ensure that things go according to plan. Don't stop the train by failing to consent the patient, order the CT or do anything like that. And, in the event that you do accidentally cause a change in the plan, be certain to load the boat!

Rule # 7: Call your consults early.

Nothing is more frustrating to get called to consult on a patient at the end of your day, when it is obvious that this was a problem that the primary service knew about hours earlier. It's bad manners and bad team work. If you know that you need Psychiatry to see a patient who has been acting up, and you are told to do this on morning rounds, this should be at the top of your to do list. Don't do all your jobs, go to the OR or whatever, and then decide to page Psychiatry at 4pm having known that you needed them to see a patient since you first rounded at 6am. There is an etiquette to residency, and you should make this a part of your routine.

Additionally, when requesting a consult, ensure that you know all the details about the patient. Anticipate what questions the service may ask you and have the answers readily available. This often includes the patient's history, hospital course, most recent vitals and most recent laboratory values.

When requesting a consult, if you are not verbally speaking to someone, it is completely unacceptable to list the reason for the consult as, "Please assess" or "Please evaluate". You must give some background history and be very specific as to why you are requesting the consult. Be sure to leave your name and contact information in a legible manner so that you may be contacted easily if necessary.

Rule # 8: One list.

Every morning, you should have a list of patient's on your service. You will use this list to make notes of the things that you need to do every day for every individual patient. Some people write down the orders then scratch them off when they've completed the task. Others make a check-box next to each order and shade it in when they've completed the list. Do whatever works for you. One thing that will not work, however, is if you have several different pieces of paper in your pocket and you're writing things all over the place. Stay organized. Organization is key to being a good intern. If Mr. Jones needs Colace, a Nephrology Consult and a CT-Scan, then write all of this down under his name on your single list.

Rule #9: White coat pockets.

A common theme to being an effective intern and resident is to stay organized. This also means to have the contents of your white coat kept in an orderly fashion. Yes you're walking around with your Pocket Medicine book or whatever, but if you rarely ever use the book, take it out of your pocket. If you have a list with you from July and it's December, chances are there is no one on that list that you are following. Take it out of your pocket, and through it away. Don't keep junk in your pockets.

At the same time, your pockets should not be empty. Identify the tools or materials that you use regularly and keep them in your pockets. For example, if you're on Urology and you know that you get a lot of calls to place foley catheters, then keep one in your pocket. You should not constantly have to search all over the floor for things that you routinely need. Stay organized and efficient. If you work in a hospital that only has paper charts, then keep admission note paper, progress note paper or whatever you use frequently in your pockets. Your goal should be to get the most done in the least amount of steps. Having said that, figure out ways to save yourself time so you can do your job quickly and efficiently.

Rule # 10: Nursing Staff.

You may be the Doctor and these are technically your patients. But at the end of the day, nobody spends more time with your patient than the nurse. Nurses can be your greatest asset. They are your eyes and ears that monitor a patient the most while you're off doing one of your many tasks. Be sure to respect your nurses and recognize that they are an invaluable part of your team. Just as you want them to let you know if things are going awry with your patient, you in turn should always keep them informed. If you're going to put a naso-gastric tube in Mr. Green, then his nurse should not find this out by walking into the room and finding him with the tube in his nose. This is your patient, but it is also the nurse's patient. Keep the nurse aware of the plan. Writing an order is one part of this, but verbally communicating the order to a nurse ensures that everyone is aware of the plan.

Your nurse can be your greatest asset. Keep them happy, and they will keep you happy. And ultimately, the patient benefits.

Rule #11: Closed loop communication.

Every member of a team should be aware of the plan on a patient. Chances are that there are several different people who are on your team looking after one patient. As such, it is important that everyone knows what is going on. Communicate with your other team members about any deviation in the plan or about anything that changes significantly with a patient. And make sure that when you tell them, they confirm with you that they've gotten your message. This is sort of a combination of load the boat and don't stop the train.

Take for example Mr. Berry who was found to be hypokalemic to 1.2 one afternoon. Having repleted the Potassium, one intern mentioned to the other that the patient had a low potassium and that he repleted it. The other intern mis-understood what was said, and went ahead and wrote a second order to replete Mr. Berry's Potassium. The nursing staff assumed that this was not an error and went ahead and gave a second dose of Potassium. The error was only discovered later that day when Mr. Berry suffered a cardiac arrhythmia secondary to potassium over-load and wound up intubated in the ICU. Clearly, this is not good patient care. Make sure that everyone is clear on the plan, at all times.

Rule # 12: All animals are equal.

Those familiar with George Orwell's "Animal Farm" may recognize this one. While it is basic human decency to treat everyone that you meet with respect, it is quite distressing to see how some people let the whole "M.D." title make them feel that they have a "G.O.D." title instead. Treat everyone that you meet with respect all the way from your Attending to the janitorial staff. This is not only the decent thing to do, but it creates a pleasant working environment of us all.

A Program Chairman I know who many actually consider to be a "God of robotic surgery" once told me this story about one of his experiences at one of the most prestigious hospitals in the country. It was the 1970s, and he was one of the first foreign medical graduates to be taken into this specialty at this institution. After a case one day, he was standing in the OR finishing up some notes on the case that he had just completed. The intern on the team who had just started a few days prior burst into the room, looked around, and started to chastise him for not cleaning up the room fast enough after surgery. The intern looked at the man's brown skin and assumed that he was a janitor. This man didn't react, but seethed with anger as he grabbed a mop and proceeded to clean the room as instructed. Later, when the second case was going on, the intern burst in, and to his chagrin, found that the "janitor" was actually the PGY-3, who was now doing the case!

Rule # 13: Systems.

Again, organization and efficiency are key to being a good intern. Having said that, if you think of a patient by systems, you will not forget anything when admitting a patient, writing orders, or more importantly, signing out to another resident about a patient. Here is a template, but the important thing is to note the headings here, as they pertain to any patient in any specialty:

NEURO: Oxycodone 5mg PO q4 PRN pain. Tylenol PRN.

CARDS: Lopressor 5mg PO TID.

LUNGS: Wean to room air.

GI: Advance diet as tolerated. Colace 100mg PO BID.

GU: NS @ 100. Flomax 0.4mg PO QD.

HEME: Venodyne boots.

ENDO: No issues.

ID: Ciprofloxacin 500mg po BID

TLD (Tubes/Lines/Drains): Foley to gravity. D/C NGT. JP drain to suction.

Rule # 14: When covering a patient, cover the patient.

There will come a time during Internship when you will be the "Float" Intern. That is, you may be on "night float" or something of that nature where you don't see a patient or group of patients during the day, but then you get sign out from a co-Intern and you are now responsible for covering or cross-covering that patient.

It is never, ever acceptable, when paged or asked a question about a patient who is under your care for you to respond, "I'm just covering right now" as an excuse for not knowing the answer. If you are responsible for a patient, then be responsible for that patient. For example, if a Nurse pages you and asks you about some CT scan or other study for a patient, you should have heard about this when you got sign-out on that patient. If you didn't get the information, then two people have failed...you and the person who signed out to you.

If someone is under you care, be sure that you know every little detail about them. A failure to do so will compromise patient care, and may result in patient detriment. And again, this falls under the concept of "Don't stop the train" as discussed earlier. If you don't know the plan for a patient under your care, regardless of how briefly you are taking care of the patient, then you haven't done your job.

Rule #15: Set your self up for success.

This rule applies in particular to a scenario where you're doing a bed-side procedure. When you have to do anything at the bedside, you should not only have all the material that you need, but you should also have them aligned in a manner that you can reach the material easily. Now this sounds simple enough, but you'll be surprised how many times you'll see people twisting and turning and reaching awkwardly for something while doing a procedure.

For example, let's say you're placing a foley catheter. You should not be twisting around to grab the lubrication, then turning to look for the foley, then turning to look for the foley bag etc. They should all be within easy reach, and should be aligned in a sequential manner based on when you are going to use them.

NOTE TEMPLATES

The following are templates to give you an idea about how to write some of the common notes that you will have to do on a daily basis. Remember, anytime you do a procedure on a patient, you should leave a note in the chart.

Also, it is of paramount importance to state what service is writing the note eg. write "Colorectal Surgery Progress Note" and not just "Progress Note". It is also of vital importance to sign your note clearly, and ensure that your pager number is legible at the end of the note so that you can be contacted readily if necessary.

The Progress Note Template

SUBJECTIVE: This reflects what the patient tells you. eg. Pain well controlled. Tolerating a diet. Ambulated three times. Passed flatus but no bowel movement reported.

OBJECTIVE: This section includes vital signs, labs, and a description of relevant physical exam eg:

98.7, 98,7 HR 72, BP 120/80, RR 18, Sat 99%on 2LNC

Ins: 1000cc

Outs: 800 (urine), 100 (NGT)

CARDS: RRR

LUNGS: CTAB

ABDOMEN: S, NT, ND

WOUNDS: CDI (Clean/dry/intact)

ASSESSMENT: eg. 57M POD (post-op day) 4 s/p laparoscopic cholecystectomy.

PLAN:

NEURO: Transition to PO pain meds (Oxycodone 5 mg PO QD) and D/C PCA.

CARDS: Re-start home Norvasc 5mg PO QD.

LUNGS: Wean to room air.

GI: Advance diet as tolerated (ADAT).

GU: HLIV (Hep-lock IV).

HEME: D/C SubQ Heparin.

ENDO: No issues.

ID: D/C IV Cipro and transition to Cipro 500 PO BID.

TLD: D/C foley.

The Clinic Note

CC (Chief Complaint): Right flank pain.

HPI (History of presenting illness): 37F presents with three day history of right flank pain. Pain radiates from right flank to her groin and is described as stabbing in nature. The pain is intermittent, rated 8/10 at it's worse and is accompanied by nausea and vomiting. There are no aggravating or relieving factors. Patient's history is notable for several kidney stones requiring surgical intervention over the past ten years. She has not had any fever at home, and, to her knowledge, she has two kidneys.

PMedHx:

1. None

ALLERGIES:

1. Sulfa drugs – hives

HOME MEDS:

1. None

PSurgHx:

1. ESWL x 5
2. Cholecystectomy
3. Hysterectomy

Social Hx:

1. 10-pack year history.
2. Denies alcohol
3. Denies drugs.

Family Hx:

1. Thyroid cancer
2. Diabetes.
3. Hypertension.

PHYSICAL EXAM:

GENERAL: Well appearing female in no acute distress.

CARDS: RRR

LUNGS: CTAB

ABDOMEN: SNTNT with no CVA tenderness.

IMAGING: KUB done 02/18/2009 notable for 9mm proximal right ureteral stone.

URINALYSIS: Notable for large blood cells, trace leukocytes and positive for nitrites.

ASSESSMENT: 37F with known history of renal stones p/w (presents with) left flank pain by three days. KUB significant for RIGHT 9mm proximal ureteral stone. Urinalysis notable for UTI.

PLAN:

Neuro: Oxycodone 5 mg po q4hours PRN pain.

CARDS: No issues

LUNGS: No issues.

GI: NPO now.

GU: NS @ 100.

HEME: VD boots.

ENDO: No issues.

ID: Cipro 400mg IV q12hours

TLD: None

LABS: CBC / Chem 7 /Coags

IMAGING: CXR, EKG.

OTHER: Consent for cystoscopy and RIGHT ureteral stent placement.

The Consult Note

Reason for consult: Gross hematuria.

HPI: 77M admitted to Medicine service (pager 64672) two days ago with shortness of breath. After foley catheter placement yesterday, the patient was noted to have dark red urine in the foley bag. Blood also noted around the penile meatus. Urology consulted to assess.

PHYSICAL EXAM:

GENERAL: Elderly appearing male in NAD. AAO x 3.

ABDOMEN: SNTND.

GU: 16F retention catheter in place with dried blood at the penile meatus. 200cc of Kool-Aid colored urine noted in the foley bag.

PROCEDURE: The 16F retention catheter was removed. With the patient supine, the area was prepped with Betadine solution then draped in the standard, sterile fashion. 10cc of UroJet (Lidocaine and lubrication) were then infused into the urethra.

A 20cc Hematuria catheter was then introduced through the urethra and into the bladder. The bladder was then flushed with approximately 500cc of saline. The urine was noted to be Kool Aid colored initially, but became light pink by the end of the procedure. Clots were noted in the irrigation fluid. The foley balloon was inflated with 30cc of normal saline.

Recommendations:
- irrigate the bladder q4hours
- keep foley in place for 5 – 10 days
- Urology to follow

CONCLUSION

Your Intern year and your Chief Resident years are probably the two years in Residency in which you will learn the most. As a result, they can be the most difficult years of your Residency. As an Intern, you have to learn to put your years of studying to practical use. But, you also have to learn to be organized and efficient. Learn to make daily check-lists for all your duties to maximize efficiency and to ensure that you don't forget to do something.

We hope that these simple rules and note templates will help you in some way, and serve as guidelines for you in this early stage of your career.

Sean L. Sawh M.D.
Francy M. Sawh M.D.

COMMON ELECTROLYTE REPLACEMENT GUIDE

POTASSIUM   **Goal: 4.0**
                                       Formula: 10meq for every 0.2 below

CALCIUM   **Goal: 10**
                                       Formula: 1gram for every 01. below

MAGNESIUM   **Goal: 1.3 – 2.1**
                                       Formula: 1 gram for every 0.1 below

URINE

Goal: 30cc / hour

Rx for low urine output: Give 1 liter bolus over 30 minutes. Reduce to 500cc if patient has a cardiac or respiratory history to avoid fluid over-load.

If urine output is low, blood pressure is low with or without accompanying tachycardia in a post-operative patient, then consider that the patient might be bleeding. Order a STAT CBC and look for a significant fall in the Hemoglobin or Hematocrit.

DAILY TASKS & OTHER SIMPLE PRINCIPLES

1. You should try to see every patient twice a day.

2. You must look at all laboratory values yourself.

3. For all Radiology studies, get in the habit of looking at the films yourself before reading the Radiologist's report. You'll be surprised at how accurate you will become with practice.

4. Anytime you do any procedure to a patient, you should leave a note in the chart.

5. Get in the habit of doing your dictations as soon as they are due.

6. Remember the old adage, "Eat when you can, sleep when you can".

7. Memorize the common telephone numbers that you have to dial every day.

8. Get to work early and give yourself a chance to look at daily notes and labs if you have a chance.

9. Never be late to work. Ever.

10. It is not acceptable to dump your work on a co-resident, junior resident, night-float or medical student.

11. When rounding in the morning, anticipate if a patient will need a dressing change and have the necessary equipment either in the room or in your pocket.

12. The Resident common room is not a dump. Clean up after yourself.

13. Walk with a snack-bar or fruit in your pocket.

14. A breath-mint will not hurt you.

15. There is such a thing as a strong chief and weak chief. Identify the former and try to emulate him or her.

16. Learn the names and doses of common pain medications, antibiotics and stool softners.

17. When admitting a patient, verbally confirm that the medical reconciliation list is up to date. This can be difficult as some patients have no idea about what meds they're taking and will often refer to their pills by color or shape eg "I take a white capsule with a line on it".

18. Keep yourself neat and presentable. A sloppy looking resident does not inspire confidence.

19. If you are unsure about a medication dosage, remember that there is an in-house Pharmacy that can help you.

20. On your day off, get some exercise.

Tips to remember when discharging a patient

1. It is inevitable that any patient admitted to your service will eventually be discharged. Start thinking about the discharge from day 1. Get the discharge note started if your particular system allows you to "tee-up" the patient to discharge them at a later date.

2. The discharge note that the patient takes home should have a detailed breakdown of every medication with the strength and frequency of each drug that the patient has to take. It is useful to include a one-liner to explain what the medication will do e.g. "For pain" or "For infection".

3. If a follow up appointment is necessary, call and make that appointment for the patient yourself. Even if the patient has to follow up with a different service, at the very least, you should provide the patient with a telephone number and not just instruct them to "make an appointment with your PCP".

4. When discharging a patient, think systematically and ensure that they have medications as needed for each system i.e Neuro, Cards, Lungs etc.

5. Make sure that the patient has a way to contact your service if they leave the Hospital and experience a problem.

Tips for Medical Students

1. Identify yourself clearly as a student. Lying to a patient is unacceptable.

2. If you are unsure about how to do something, stop and ask someone.

3. Observe the resident's daily tasks and see if there is anything that you can do to make their life easier e.g. write the Progress Note or check the labs if you know that they are pending.

4. If you see a medication that is unfamiliar to you, write down the name and look it up later on.

5. If you have the opportunity to see a procedure, regardless of how simple, go see it so that you can do it the next time.

6. Do every procedure that you can before graduating. The first time that you place a Naso-Gastric tube or remove a central line should not be when you are an Intern. Try to do this at least once as a student and it will make your Internship just a little bit easier.

7. Become proficient at phlebotomy. You WILL take blood as an Intern at some point.

8. Get BCLS and ACLS certified.

9. If the residents are looking at a CT/ XRAY/Ultrasound, and you can't see what they're referring to, just ask. You are a student. Your job is to learn.

10. Learn to write efficient patient notes. Read the residents notes and tailor your notes to match. Eventually, you will learn to separate the important information from the fluff.

11. If you are following a patient, you should know him as well as the resident.

12. Get in the habit of coming up with your own daily plan when you see a patient and compare it to what the plan is when you hear the residents talk about the patient.

13. Make yourself a part of the team, but at the same time, don't get in the way or slow down the team.

BLANK PAGE

30

BLANK PAGE

BLANK PAGE

www.ingramcontent.com/pod-product-compliance
Lightning Source LLC
Chambersburg PA
CBHW071559170526
45166CB00004B/1720